Intermittent Fasting

The Beginner's Guide

By PROSENCE

Respective authors own all copyrights not held by the publisher.

The information herein is offered for informational purposes solely, and is universal as so. The presentation of the information is without contract or any type of guarantee assurance.

The trademarks that are used are without any consent, and the publication of the trademark is without permission or backing by the trademark owner. All trademarks and brands within this book are for clarifying purposes only and are the owned by the owners themselves, not affiliated with this document.

ABOUT PROSENCE
Our Mission

We are dedicated to guiding, motivating and providing the tools necessary to transform people into the best version of themselves. Our goal is to empower men and women across the globe to realize that physical and mental fitness are not a short-term solution, but a lifetime choice- and to actualize what they have come to understand into a daily routine. We invite you to discover this process for yourself as you join us in the exploration of science-based knowledge that can lead to better health, greater fulfilment and astonishing vitality.

Who is Prosence?

Prosence is led by Antonio Mazzotta, a strapping 28-year-old Italian health enthusiast who resides in Switzerland. He's a self-described "Mr. Nice Guy" who, (despite a powerful love for his mamma's pasta and pizza), has developed a life dedicated to health and fitness. Now, he strives to share his secrets with the world.

Antonio discovered his passion for health and fitness 7 years ago and has never looked back! Days are filled with working new routines at his gym, training hard, meeting like-minded people and, dear to his heart, teaching weight training, dieting, and healthy lifestyle choices to his valued clients. Job one is helping people to achieve their overall fitness goals, including providing a gain in endurance and a new (sustainable) vitality.

He and his team fight to counter the preponderance of bad information that proliferates the Internet, being driven by offering people a safe yet powerful path to vibrant, brilliant health. In short, *Prosence* is fervently dedicated to the motivation, inspiration and education of people via the dissemination of the real science-based information they need to get into great shape and to stay healthy for a lifetime.

Discover today how we can help you to grow into what you were meant to be and to embrace life to the fullest with newly realized passion!

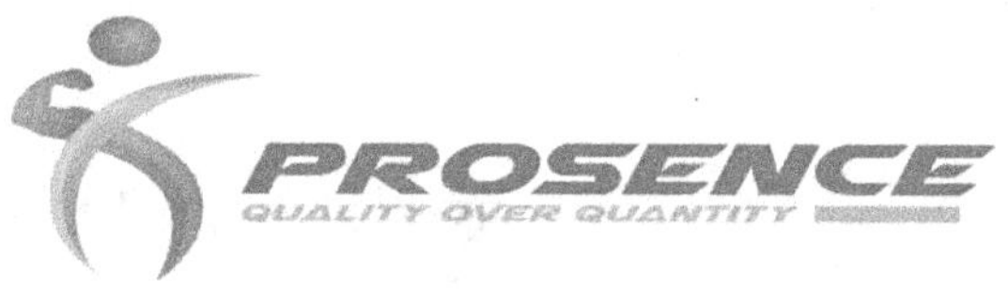

Table of Contents

Introduction

I want to thank you and congratulate you for purchasing the book, "Intermittent Fasting: *The Beginner's Guide.*"

Do you want to lose weight and improve your overall health? Does the thought of counting calories make you wary of dieting? Wouldn't it be wonderful if you could achieve your health and weight loss goals without counting calories? Well, if your answer is yes to the above-mentioned questions, then in such a case intermittent fasting is the diet that you have been looking for.

Fasting is not a new concept, and it has been around since time immemorial. Intermittent fasting is a simple variation of fasting, and it is quite helpful. This dieting protocol oscillates between periods of fasting and eating.

In this book, you will learn what intermittent fasting is all about, various health benefits it offers, the most popular forms of intermittent fasting, research that supports the health benefits of this diet, gaining muscle while on this diet, and read common FAQs about this diet together with a step-by-step plan for getting started with this diet.

Intermittent fasting is a very simple concept, and by making a couple of changes to your eating habits, you can reap all the benefits this diet offers. Do you want to learn more about this fascinating diet? Then let us get started without further ado.

Thanks again for purchasing this book. I hope you enjoy it!

Chapter 1
What is Intermittent Fasting?

The latest trend that has taken the world of fitness by a storm is intermittent fasting. This dieting protocol involves the oscillation between periods of fasting and eating. In this chapter, you will learn what intermittent fasting is all about.

Intermittent fasting is all about alternating between periods of eating and fasting. There are no dietary restrictions according to this diet. It focuses on when you eat instead of what you eat. There are different variations of this diet and it can be easily customized to suit your personal needs. Fasting certainly isn't a new concept and people usually fast for health or spiritual reasons. Or at times even the lack of food can be a cause. There are different religions like Buddhism, Hinduism, Islam and Christianity that prescribe fasting. Did you know that we are all used to fasting daily? Yes, take a moment and think about it. You are effectively fasting while sleeping, aren't you? Intermittent fasting is a mere extension of this fasting period. If you aren't used to having your breakfast and have your first meal at noon and the last one at 8 in the evening, you are unconsciously following a pattern of intermittent fasting. Yes, it actually is as simple as that. While following any pattern of intermittent fasting, you just need to make sure that you are eating only during your feeding window. Fasting is quite easy and if you are worried about feeling hungry, that can be tackled easily. While fasting, you can have any calorie-free beverage like green tea or black coffee without worrying about breaking your fast.

There isn't anything unnatural about fasting as our bodies are designed in a manner that we can survive even without consuming food for a prolonged period. Several processes in your bodies change when you start fasting. The level of blood sugar and insulin decrease while there is an increase in the production of the growth hormone. Some might follow it for the weight loss benefits it offers and others for the metabolic benefits of intermittent fasting.

There are different intermittent fasting protocols and depending on your lifestyle; you can select a method that suits your needs.

16/8 Protocol

In this method, you will fast for 16 hours, and the eating window is restricted to just 8 hours. So, if you start your fast at 8 pm, then you can break your fast at 12 pm the next day. Lunch will be your first meal, and your last meal should be before 8 pm. And the cycle will start again. Since we don't get any nutrients while sleeping, it makes sense to include the time spent sleeping as a part of the 16 hours.

18/6 Protocol

This is similar to the 16/8 protocol except that you only have 6 hours during which you can eat. If you start fasting at 8 pm, you will have to fast until 2 pm on the following day. Your feeding window extends till 8 pm, and then the cycle starts again.

1 Day Feast/1 Day Fast

This method is self-explanatory. You will have to fast on every alternate day. If you are eating like you usually do on Monday, then you will have to fast on Tuesday, and break your fast on Wednesday and so on.

The Warrior Diet

This is like the 16/8 protocol, and you will have to fast daily. However, your feeding window is restricted to just 4 hours at night. You will have to fast the entire day and have a huge meal at night. You might be wondering why you would do this. The answer given by the proponents of this method is that, by doing this, hormone production in the body is optimized and excess fat burnt, particularly if you reduce your intake of carbohydrates.

5/2 Diet

In this method of intermittent fasting, you eat, as usual, for three days then have a fasting day followed by two days of feasting followed by another fasting day after which the cycle repeats. On fasting days, you can eat food with a caloric content of about 500-600 calories.

Perhaps the most liberal of all intermittent fasting protocols is the Anything Goes Method. Eat only when your body tells you that you need food. Eat only when hunger strikes you and not because you have to. This is extremely simple. If you are busy at work and don't feel like eating, you simply need to skip a meal. That's about it.

Chapter 2
24-hour Fasting

The 24-hour fasting protocol is self-explanatory, isn't it? As the name suggests, you will need to fast for 24 hours. You can fast once or twice a week depending on your schedule and your needs. This method was popularized by Brad Pilon, a fitness expert. It is a very simple fasting protocol, and you don't have to do much. If you had your dinner at 8 pm, then you will be required to fast until the same time on the following day. If you start fasting at 8 pm, then the fast will extend until 8 pm on the consecutive day. Then your eating window will start from 8 pm to 8 pm on the following day.

It is quite simple. You can decide how you want to fast. The aim is to fast for 24-hours at a stretch. Depending on your convenience you can select your fasting schedule. You can also fast from breakfast on a given day till breakfast time on the following day. You aren't allowed to consume any solid food, but you can have calorie-free beverages like green tea, black coffee, other herbal teas, and lots of water. If you are following this dieting protocol with the intention of losing weight, then make sure that during your eating window you are having healthy food and aren't having any junk food. It might seem a little intimidating, at least initially. Well, you don't have to worry. Fasting isn't difficult. You can start by following a simpler intermittent fasting protocol like the 16/8 method before moving on to the 24-hour fasting method. Make sure that you aren't fasting on two consecutive days. You can do this twice or thrice in a week depending on your weight loss goals.

Keep yourself busy on your fasting days. When you don't have any free time, then you won't think about food. Indulge in activities that will keep you occupied. Have plenty of water and keep your body fully hydrated at all times. Water also helps in making you feel full. Plan your week in such a way that your fasting days don't clash with any of your social obligations. You don't have to compromise on your social life for the sake of this diet. It just requires a little bit of planning. This method is quite helpful and very simple to follow.

Sunday	Monday	Tuesday	Wednesday	Thursday	Friday	Saturday
Eat normally	Start fasting after dinner. Around 8pm in the night	Fast until 8pm in the night	Eat normally	Start fasting after dinner. Around 8pm in the night	Fast until 8pm in the night	Eat normally

Chapter 3
16/8 Fasting

According to this method, you will need to fast for 16 hours daily. The eating window is restricted to 8 hours every day. You can squeeze in two or three small meals within this eating window. This method of intermittent fasting is also known as Leangains, and a fitness expert named Martin Berkhan popularized it. It could be something as simple as skipping breakfast and not snacking on anything before lunch and then directly having your dinner at night. Your first meal can be at 12 noon instead of a morning breakfast, and then your last meal can be at 8 pm in the evening.

The fasting period according to this method extends to 16 hours. It is usually advised that women shouldn't fast for more than 14-15 hours per day. If you are used to waking up early and exercising in the morning, then you can adjust this method so that it fits in your schedule quite easily. You can have your breakfast and lunch and skip dinner. Your first meal can be at 10 am in the morning and your last meal at 6 pm in the evening.

The feeding window extends to 8 hours and the rest of the day would go away in fasting. Plan your schedule in such a manner that your sleeping period is included within the 16 hours that you have to fast. You cannot feel hungry if you are sleeping, can you? However, you aren't much of a breakfast eater and are used to skipping your breakfast already, then in such a case, this method would work well for you. And you wouldn't have to make any changes to your daily schedule. You can have water, coffee, and other beverages that don't have any calories in it while you are fasting. It is important that you stay away from all forms of junk food and eat healthy during the fast. This diet won't work out if you binge on foods that have a high caloric value. It will be easier to stick to intermittent fasting if you consume low-calorie meals.

Timings	Sunday	Monday	Tuesday	Wednesday	Thursday	Friday	Saturday
Midnight	Sleeping and fasting	Sleeping and fasting	Sleeping and fasting	Sleeping and fasting	Sleeping and fasting	Sleeping and fasting	Sleeping and fasting
4 am	Sleeping and fasting	Sleeping and fasting	Sleeping and fasting	Sleeping and fasting	Sleeping and fasting	Sleeping and fasting	Sleeping and fasting
8 am	Fasting	Fasting	Fasting	Fasting	Fasting	Fasting	Fasting
Till Noon	Fasting	Fasting	Fasting	Fasting	Fasting	Fasting	Fasting

4 pm	Break the fast after noon	Break the fast after noon	Break the fast after noon	Break the fast after noon	Break the fast after noon	Break the fast after noon	Break the fast after noon
8 pm	Feeding window	Feeding window	Feeding window	Feeding window	Feeding window	Feeding window	Feeding window
Midnight	Fasting period	Fasting period	Fasting period	Fasting period	Fasting period	Fasting period	Fasting period

Chapter 4
The Truth About Breakfast

Do you want to speed up the process of weight loss and enable your body to burn fat efficiently? Then skipping your breakfast will do the trick. Human physiology is based on the feast-famine pattern of eating; the basic hunter-gatherer nature of the homosapien ancestors is instilled in us. We live in the modern world where there is no dearth of food, but our bodies haven't had much time to get adapted to this change. This constant dilemma between the modern society and our basic physiology isn't a new one. It is not a good idea to ignore this science of ours. Instead, you should understand it so that you can make the most of it and improve the overall metabolism of your body.

It is a popular belief that the most important meal of the day is the breakfast. Almost all the weight-loss regimes recommend the consumption of a hearty breakfast. So, where does this basic idea arise? There is another popular myth that claims that skipping breakfast is directly related to obesity. Well, how can you put on weight while restricting your calorie intake? Sounds absurd, doesn't it? No scientific research supports this claim. So, it is nothing more than a myth and skipping breakfast will not make you fat. In fact, a research that was published in The American Journal of Clinical Nutrition (2014) showed no effect from either eating or skipping breakfast on weight loss.

Always listen to your body when it comes to consumption of food. Eat only when you are hungry, and your body will tell you when it needs food. If you aren't hungry in the morning, then skip your breakfast. It is perfectly normal to skip your breakfast, and a lot of people do this. "Breakfast is the most important meal of the day" is nothing but a myth.

Did you ever wonder why you don't feel hungry in the morning? The circadian system is responsible for keeping us in sync with the 24-hour day and our response to light and darkness. This system also influences your hormones, body temperature, and the process of digestion. The circadian system regulates your hunger and appetite and is responsible for the lack of hunger in the morning and the hunger pangs you experience in the evening. Even if you fast for the whole night, you will not feel hungry in the morning, and the circadian system is responsible for it.

Your body will not burn fat if there is a constant supply of glycogen. If you eat five to six meals daily, you will not burn any fat. The body can easily access glucose since it is readily available. If you want your body to burn fat, then you can accomplish this by restricting your food intake. The food that you consume is converted into glucose, and the excess glucose is stored in the form of fat in the body. When you restrict your consumption of food by fasting for prolonged periods of time, your body will reach into its fat stores for providing energy. You can optimize this by postponing the first meal of the day, and intermittent fasting helps with this. People tend to believe that our body requires a constant supply of glucose and end up eating after every couple of hours. This might be true if you have a low sugar level or have diabetes. If you are a healthy individual, then you certainly don't need to keep eating after every three or four hours. If you keep feeding your body all the time, it simply develops resistance towards insulin and causes unnecessary health problems.

The most popular intermittent fasting protocol is the one that recommends the skipping of breakfast. While sleeping your body produces certain hormones that break down the fat that's stored in the body. This provides your body with a burst of energy as soon as you wake up in the morning. This spurt of energy will keep you going for a couple of hours at least. So, your body doesn't necessarily require breakfast, and by skipping it, you aren't harming yourself.

Chapter 5
What Does the Research Say?

Intermittent fasting is a pattern of eating that alternates between periods of eating and fasting. In this chapter, let us take a look at the different health benefits that this dieting protocol offers according to scientific research.

Changes the functioning of cells

When you restrict your calorie intake while fasting, several changes take place in your body. For instance, cellular repair takes place, and there are changes in the levels of certain hormones that help in accessing the stored fat in the body. The insulin levels decrease in the body, and this helps in burning stored fat for generating energy. There is also a spike in the production of growth hormone. This hormone is responsible for facilitating the burning of fat and muscle gain. Cellular repair also starts, and this includes the process of removal of accumulated wastes in the body. The same was proved by a study that was published in The Journal of Clinical Investigation- The American Society for Clinical Investigation.

(https://www.ncbi.nlm.nih.gov/pmc/articles/PMC329619/)

Helps in losing weight loss and belly fat

The main reason why a lot of people opt for this diet is that it helps in weight loss. Intermittent fasting helps in weight loss by reducing your calorie intake. Unless you try and compensate for this by eating more during your eating window, you are bound to lose weight. In a study that was conducted by the University of Aberdeen Rowett Institute of Nutrition and Health, Aberdeen, Scotland, UK it was discovered that intermittent fasting also helps in producing a higher level of growth hormone and lower levels of insulin that enable the body to burn fat for generating energy. This is the reason why there is a spike in your metabolic rate when you are following the protocols of intermittent fasting. Intermittent fasting assists weight loss by reducing your calorie intake and boosting your metabolism. It also helps in the build-up of lean muscle.

(https://www.ncbi.nlm.nih.gov/pubmed/25540982)

Reduces the risk of type-2 diabetes

One of the major health problems these days is type-2 diabetes, and this condition can be effectively managed by following intermittent fasting protocols. A high level of blood sugar makes your body resistant to insulin. Insulin helps in reducing the blood sugar levels, and when the body becomes resistant to this, the blood sugar simply increases. In a research that was conducted by Division of Endocrinology, Department of Medicine, the University of Illinois at Chicago, Chicago it was recorded that intermittent fasting helps in reducing the body's resistance towards insulin and helps in regulating blood sugar levels.

(http://www.sciencedirect.com/science/article/pii/S193152441 400200X)

It helps in reducing inflammation

Inflammation is the leading cause of several chronic health conditions. This occurs when unstable molecules react with other useful molecules like protein or DNA and damage them in the process. Several studies show that intermittent fasting can successfully improve the body's resistance towards oxidative stress.

(https://www.hindawi.com/journals/bmri/2014/761264/)

Promotes heart's health

One of the terrible problems plaguing humanity is cardiovascular disease. Most of the health markers are related to an increase or decrease in the risk associated to heart diseases. Intermittent fasting helps in improving various risk factors like blood pressure, good cholesterol, level of triglycerides, and even control the levels of blood sugar. However, most of the data supporting these claims have been collected from animal studies. Department of Kinesiology and Nutrition, the University of Illinois at Chicago, Chicago, IL 60612, USA. varady@uic.edu

(https://www.ncbi.nlm.nih.gov/pubmed/19793855)

Chapter 6
Frequency of Fasting

Intermittent fasting is a pattern of eating that oscillates between periods of eating and fasting. There are a lot of myths about this method of fasting. In this chapter, let us debunk the most popular misconceptions that exist about fasting, snacking, and the frequency of eating.

Skipping breakfast will make you gain weight

In the previous chapter, you learned why breakfast isn't as important as people claim it to be. It might be considered to be the most important meal of the day, but it isn't, and that notion is just a myth. People believe that skipping breakfast leads to excessive hunger and weight gain. No scientific studies or research supports this claim. Skipping breakfast won't make you fat, and you can do so quite safely without any fear. You can fast for 16 to 24 hours at a stretch without worrying about the functioning of your body. Your body knows what's best for it; trust your body.

Your metabolism improves when you eat frequently

It is a popular myth that eating frequently helps in improving your metabolism. Eating small meals does not improve your body's ability to burn calories. Yes, your body does need some energy to digest and assimilate the food you consume. This is referred to as the thermic effect of food, and it accounts for about 20-30% of total calories from protein, 5-10% from carbs and about 3% from fats. On an average, the thermic effect of food accounts for 10% of the total calories you consume. You need to take into consideration the total calories you consume and not the number of meals you eat. You don't need to keep eating constantly. For instance, if you have three meals of 1000 calories each the thermic effect would be 300 calories, and it will be the same if you have six meals of 500 calories each. So, you can fast for prolonged periods of time and not worry about slowing down your body's metabolism.

Eating frequently helps in keeping hunger at bay

People believe that snacking constantly helps in keeping hunger at bay and reduces the chances of excessive hunger. Frequent meals will obviously leave you feeling full, but you don't have to do this. If you want to reduce your cravings and keep hunger at bay, then you need to make sure that you are filling yourself up with the right kind of food. Your meals should contain high amounts of fiber, protein, and healthy fats instead of carbs. A meal that's rich in carbs will make you feel hungry soon and make you want to eat more food. Consuming carbs makes you crave for carbs. So, a balanced meal is the key to reducing your hunger. You don't have to worry about hunger pangs while following the protocols of intermittent fasting.

Small meals assist in weight loss

Like mentioned earlier, frequent meals don't help in boosting your metabolism. Small meals won't do your body any good, and they certainly don't help in weight loss. Eating frequently has the opposite of the desired effect. You can fast for an entire day without worrying about your body metabolism. There won't be a change in your energy levels if you keep snacking regularly. If you are worried that fasting leads to weight gain, you can lay those fears to rest. In fact, your body will start burning its reserves of fat for providing energy if you restrict the supply of glucose.

The brain needs glucose constantly

Yes, the brain does need glucose to function. This doesn't mean that you need to keep consuming carbs every couple of hours for our brain to keep functioning. It certainly won't stop functioning if you don't eat anything for an extended period. This misconception is due to the assumption that the brain needs glucose for functioning. Even if you restrict the consumption of food, your body can burn fats and produce energy that will keep your body going. Your body starts producing glucose that's necessary by a process known as gluconeogenesis. There is a reserve of glucose in the body, and your liver breaks this down to supply glucose that is essential for the functioning of your brain. Even during the 24-hour format of fasting, your brain will function, and you don't have to worry about that. The dietary fats present in the body will be broken down into ketones by the liver for supplying the necessary energy your body needs. Ketones help in the functioning of the brain. Think about this from an evolutionary point of view. Human beings should have become extinct a long time ago if carbs were the only way for our survival. However, if an individual has hypoglycemia, then they will need to snack after every couple of hours if they don't want to get sick.

Eating often is necessary for good health

Being in a constantly fed state isn't natural for the human body. During evolution, humans had to endure periods of starvation. If eating often were essential for survival, then the human race would have been wiped out a long time ago. In fact, fasting helps in inducing cellular repair by kickstarting the process of autophagy. This helps in protecting against diseases like

Alzheimer's and even certain types of cancers. Fasting is quite beneficial for the system, and it helps in cleansing the system by eliminating the build-up of toxins in the body. Snacking often has certain disadvantages as well. Frequent meals increase your calorie intake and also lead to a build-up of fatty cells in the liver. This doesn't do your body any good.

Fasting shift your body into "starvation mode"

A popular argument against intermittent fasting is that it puts your body in starvation mode. While fasting, the body assumes that its starving, and therefore shuts down its metabolism and prevents the burning of fat for producing energy. Long-term weight loss reduces the calories you burn, and that's what starvation mode is. However, this is bound to happen regardless of the dieting protocol you follow. Short-term fasting helps to speed up the metabolic function of the body. The increase in the levels of noradrenaline in the body increases the breaking down of the fat cells and thereby boosts the metabolism as well. Fasting for up to 48 hours helps in boosting the metabolism, but anything more than this reverses this effect. You can fast as long as you follow a sensible fasting protocol.

You will lose muscle while fasting

Once again, it is nothing more than a misconception that fasting leads to muscle loss. Fasting leads to fat loss and nothing else. In fact, intermittent fasting helps in increasing the build-up of lean muscle, and when coupled with the right exercises, it helps in building muscle. Continuous calorie restriction for days together leads to the loss of muscle. However, this isn't the case with intermittent fasting, and you don't have to worry about losing muscle. You will learn more about building muscle in the coming chapters.

It is bad for your health

Some believe that fasting is harmful. Intermittent fasting has several health benefits, and scientific research can back these claims. So, thinking that fasting is bad for overall well being is nothing but a myth, and it shouldn't be taken seriously. In the previous chapter, the different health benefits of intermittent fasting and the research that backs those claims have been explained in great detail.

Intermittent fasting leads to overeating

Some claim that intermittent fasting doesn't result in weight loss and it instead leads to overeating. After a fast, your consumption of food might be slightly higher. But this wears off quite quickly. Once your body gets acclimatized to prolonged periods of fasting, your calorie intake will start decreasing. You won't try to compensate for your fasting period by eating more during your eating window. Your body will slowly get used to fasting, and you certainly don't have to worry about putting on weight.

Fasting certainly isn't bad for you, and it can help in improving your overall health. Depending on the intermittent fasting protocol that you opt for, your fasting schedule would change. You don't have to worry about the frequency of fasting since your body will get the sufficient nutrients it needs for functioning properly.

Chapter 7
Can you Still Gain Muscle and Weight while Fasting?

Did you know that you could manage to gain weight and build muscle while following intermittent fasting protocols? In fact, most of the weight that you gain will be in the form of muscle. Doesn't that sound fantastic? Well, read on to learn more about it. This happens because intermittent fasting isn't necessarily about the reduction in your daily calorie intake- though that would be the case if your main reason for picking this dieting method is shedding excess body fat- instead, it is about reducing the frequency of your meals. In other words, if you are interested in building muscle while following intermittent fasting, then you should focus on increasing your daily calorie intake during the feeding window.

The reason why people naturally equate intermittent fasting with fat or weight loss is that the natural tendency is to eat fewer calories when you cut out a meal or two daily. But, as I mentioned earlier, intermittent fasting is more about meal frequency and spacing, not total calories. So to build muscle, you simply need to consume more calories daily, and you can still do that even if you limit your eating frequency or period. Simply consume all your daily caloric needs within the remaining number of meals or eating period that you have. Apart from having to go on an empty stomach for longer, the other challenge would be to eat more than the usual amount of food per meal or within your eating window. As such, you can still gain muscle, if so desired, while on an intermittent fast. Remember Hugh Jackman? Right!

As a result, more and more people are starting to become curious about intermittent fasting in general and in the different protocols in particular. Choosing a particular protocol depends on one's lifestyle and daily schedule. Some have more time to follow the more time-consuming rules while others have less so, the simpler but harder protocols may be just what the nutritionist and trainer ordered for them. More than the schedule, another aspect of lifestyle is religion. Muslims, for example, are required to fast daily from 5 in the morning to 7 in the evening during Ramadan.

Regardless of your circumstances, you can practice intermittent fasting and incorporate a great workout regimen that will allow you to build more muscle and eventually, reduce body fat. This is because muscle cells are metabolically active, i.e., the more of it you have, the faster your metabolism becomes.

The following are guidelines to help you successfully build muscle while fasting intermittently.

The Later, The Better

If, like the Muslims, you choose a specific period of fasting daily like the Ramadan-prescribed 5 a.m. to 7 p.m. schedule, you'd be well off to schedule your exercise or workout sessions late in the evening or even early morning. Doing so helps you to get your nutrients in before and after working out, especially if you're talking about lifting weights. You can have your first meal at 7 p.m. and an hour or two after, hit the weights. Eat a recovery meal before hitting the sack say at 10 p.m. Then you can wake up before 5 a.m. to have another meal to power you through the rest of the day so by the time 5 a.m. rolls in, you've already replenished much-needed nutrients and are fully charged for the day.

Post Workout

In attempting to build muscle while fasting intermittently, the wisest way for you to apportion your daily calories is by putting the biggest chunk of your calories on your post-workout meal. The reason for this is post-workout recovery and calories consumed during the 3-hour golden post-workout window tend to be used more efficiently by the body, e.g., for building muscle instead of being stored as fat.

That being said, you'll need to figure out just how many calories you need to build muscle and consume about 20% of that before exercising or working out. Take in a good mixture of carbs and protein. Then as soon as you end your workout, consume about 60% of your calories right after your workout and before hitting the sack. If it's too much for you, consider spreading it out over 2 to 3 meals within the next 2 to 4 hours before hitting the sack.

Taking in 60% of your daily caloric requirements may seem too much to take in a relatively short span of time, and frankly, it can be intimidating. If you find that after several days you're still having a hard time doing so, then consider eating foods that are calorie dense, i.e., contain more calories per gram such as dried fruits, red meat, bagels and raw oats, among others, for you to meet the requirement. Since calorie dense foods have packed significantly more calories, you can eat less in terms of volume and still meet your 60% target. Just keep it to at most 15% of total daily calories. And because fat is the most calorie dense among the three major macronutrients at nine calories per gram compared to only four calories per gram each for carbs and protein, high-fat foods can be a good way to reduce the volume of food you need without scrimping on calories.

Eat As Soon As You Wake Up

Lastly, it's best that you eat something right after your natural waking up time when fasting intermittently. If you're sticking to the 5 a.m. to 7 p.m. fasting period Ramadan-style, it means making sure you eat something before 5 a.m. In particular, go for a slow-digesting protein that can help you feel fuller for longer and help keep your body in an anabolic state, i.e., muscle building state, for longer during the day even without eating. These food items include red meat and cottage cheese, which should make up the remaining 20% of your daily caloric requirements.

While it's not a bad idea to throw in some carbs into the meal, limit the amount so that you get at least 35% of your daily protein-calorie requirements from this meal, which is crucial to maintaining an anabolic state throughout the day. Do this with the goal of consuming only 20% of your total daily caloric requirements for this meal.

Don't Scrimp On The Calories

If you're going relatively higher intensity or volume workout sessions, just make sure you consume enough calories to power such workouts. While you can sustain such workouts with low calories and intermittent fasting, it won't be long before it catches up with you and your burnout. It's just not possible because over time, your glycogen stores will be depleted and your workouts and recovery will be severely compromised. As such, you'll need to learn to eat more food within a smaller period and less eating frequency to ensure you get enough calories to build muscle. Over time, you'll adjust to it, and it'll feel natural to you.

Chapter 8
How to get Started Today

Well, you have learned what intermittent fasting is all about. Now, all that's left for you to do is to get started with this diet. Intermittent fasting isn't just a dieting protocol but it is a way of living, and it is quite efficient in the long run for marinating your weight loss and overall health as well. Intermittent fasting will help you in shedding all those extra kilos that you have meant to get rid of. In this chapter, you will learn about the different steps that you can make use of for getting started with this diet. By following the simple steps mentioned in this chapter, intermittent fasting will not seem intimidating anymore.

Step 1: Selecting the intermittent fasting protocol

There are different intermittent fasting protocols to choose from. Intermittent fasting is one of the most versatile dieting protocols and depending upon your lifestyle, personality and goals; you can select a method of fasting that suits you perfectly.

Select a method that will fit perfectly into your life. If you are used to waking up early in the morning and enjoy working out in the morning, then in such a case, you can select the 16/8 dieting protocol where your first meal can be at 10 a.m. and the last meal at 4 p.m. You can follow the same dieting protocol if you are used to skipping your breakfast. If that's the case, then your first meal can be at noon and your last meal at 8 p.m. If you can go through the day without eating, then you can follow the warrior diet. If you like the idea of fasting on alternate days, then the eat-stop-eat protocol would suit your needs.

Step 2: Do plenty of research

Go through the information that's been provided in this book for selecting a method that suits your needs. Set goals for yourself before you consider the dieting method you want to select. Take into consideration your lifestyle and your goals; you can select an intermittent fasting protocol that suits your needs. Check your priorities and see which of the intermittent methods will suit your need. Once you know what your goals are, do plenty of research so that you select the right fasting protocol. If you want, you can try all the different methods to see which of these methods works the best for you. If you are interested in reducing your body fat and increasing your muscle mass, then you can opt for the LeanGains method.

Step 3: Find the necessary tools

There are plenty of mobile applications to choose from. There are free and paid apps that can help you in tracking your progress and help you along the way. Intermittent fasting is a method of trial and error. One method might work for some and something else for others. So, you can download an application that will help you in tracking the most efficient way. If you are more old school, then you can maintain a food journal for tracking your progress.

Step 4: Starting the transition

Unless you are an all or nothing sort of a person, starting this diet can be slightly difficult. If you aren't used to fasting, then going for prolonged periods of time without food will seem a little daunting. Well, you can lay your fears to rest. You just need some time to condition your body to this form of dieting and nothing else. You can start with a relatively simpler method of fasting before taking up something that is slightly more difficult. For instance, you can start with the 16/8 method. Or an even easier thing to do would be to transition yourself into one of the dieting protocols slowly. For instance, you can start by slowly increasing the time between your meals and while eating, make sure that you are consuming those foods that will make you feel fuller for longer. If you are used to having three meals a day and a couple of snacks between the meals, then you can start by eliminating these snacks. Then you can go ahead and decrease the number of meals you have. Or you could just start following any of the variations of this diet, and your body will automatically get used to it within a week or two.

Step 5: Finding the necessary support

It would also be helpful if you could start the diet with a partner. It could be your friend, your spouse or even a family member. You can go through the diet with them. Each can use the other as a coach and a support system. You can fast together and exercise together. Whenever you feel like giving up, there would be someone else to keep you motivated and make sure that you are on the right track. It is simpler to shop for groceries and plan your meals when you have company.

Step 6: Toning down your workouts

Usually, potency needs minimalism. For instance, the strength of coffee or even an alcoholic drink reduces when you dilute it with water. The efficiency of your workouts while following any of the intermittent fasting methods will follow suit if you train too much. What does overtraining look like in this context? Training too hard for too long. Exerting yourself when you are fasting will just burn you out, and you can even injure yourself or fall sick during this process. Even at the right intensity, pushing yourself too hard for a prolonged period won't do you any good, and you can effectively retard your progress. Draw up an exercise schedule for yourself and follow it. You can work on different muscle groups on different days of the week.

A good way to focus your training is to prioritize compound exercises, i.e., those that involve the most number of the main muscle groups to execute the movements. Another way of prioritizing your exercise is to go for those that utilize the biggest muscle groups, particularly legs and bag. Why? The bigger the muscles, the more calories are required to contract them. That's why doing 1,000 crunches aren't enough to get you ripped but running daily for at least 30 minutes, which involves the biggest muscle group that's the legs, can help you do so.

Step 7: Following delayed gratification

Delayed gratification is a brilliant technique to make use of. It works extremely well with intermittent fasting. If your co-workers at your workplace have got some yummy sweet treats to work and you are extremely hungry, your mind will tell you to give in. When the hunger pang strikes you, even a bowl of frosted cereal with cold milk seems quite appetizing. All that you will need to tell yourself is that you can eat all that, but not at the given point of time. You can even write down the list of foods that you had denied yourself. This will not only help you in staying focused, but it will also stop your mind from obsessing over the foods that you cannot eat.

Step 8: Protein should be a priority

Always make sure that you are having your proteins and complex carbs before anything else. You might have something sweet or oily on your eating list. However, eating those before anything else can prove to be quite problematic. If you consume such items first, you will end up overeating. Not only are these food items rich in calories and the amount of nutrients is minimal. All that you will end up with is a tummy ache. It will be helpful if you have planned your meals and make sure that it has got sufficient protein and complex carbohydrates in it. It is likely that you will start craving for these things by the time your feeding window approaches. Make sure that you fill yourself up with grilled chicken, lentils, or any other form of proteins, and some healthy vegetables. You can include a few carbs in the form of sweet potatoes, potatoes, a serving of rice, or something starchy. After you have had all this, there will be little or no space left for any form of junk food. Your hunger will force you to fill yourself up with the good stuff, and you won't binge on unhealthy junk.

Step 9: Taking a "before" photograph

Before you get started with intermittent fasting, the one thing that you need to do would be to take a picture of yourself. This would be the "before" photograph. This will help you in getting started with the diet. If you follow the intermittent fasting protocols, you will find the motivation you need to get through. You can gauge your progress by comparing yourself to the image. This will make you want to keep going. Your weight might not reduce immediately, but you can slowly see the fat giving way to lean muscle.

Step 10: Things to keep in mind

If you are just getting started with intermittent fasting or you want to give this diet a go, you will need to remember one important thing. The initial phase of this diet is the hardest to get through. The initial two weeks are the toughest, and after that, it does get easier. This is the toughest time since your body is just getting used to the fasting schedule. You will slowly start to gain control over your cravings, hunger pangs, and your appetite too. It can take anywhere from a few days to a few weeks for your body to get acclimatized to the diet. So, give yourself some time and let your body get used to the diet.

Chapter 9
FAQ

In this chapter, all the common FAQs about intermittent fasting have been answered.

Will fasting lead to an increase in fat storage? Will the body enter into starvation mode?

If you keep eating after every two or three hours from the time you wake up until you go to sleep at night, you are actually suppressing the process of burning fat. Your body never gets a chance to burn anything else apart from all the food that you are constantly consuming, and it makes fat loss quite difficult. Fasting helps in reducing your insulin levels, and this is useful for promoting lipolysis. Lipolysis is the process through which your body starts burning all the stored fat. When you are fasting, your body burns fat. When you eat, your body is busy breaking down the food you are consuming. So, you don't have to worry about your metabolism slowing down, and your body does not enter into a starvation mode.

Is it necessary to eat every couple of hours to maintain stable blood sugar levels?

No. Unless you have hypoglycemia, you don't have to worry about feeling light-headed if you don't eat every couple of hours. Skipping breakfast won't do you any harm. As mentioned in the earlier chapter, this is nothing more than a myth that you needn't worry about. Our bodies have been designed in such a way that we can go on for a couple of days without worrying about running out of fuel to survive.

What to eat while following this diet?

This diet doesn't prescribe any dietary restrictions per se. You need to be mindful of when you are eating and not what you are eating while following any of the intermittent dieting protocols. However, this doesn't mean that you fast for 16 hours in a day and then fill yourself up with all sorts of processed junk food. Doing this will simply defeat the purpose of dieting. There are no dietary restrictions, and you don't have to count calories, but this doesn't mean that you eat food that will promote weight gain. Have a well-balanced meal that's full of the necessary nutrients and dietary fiber that will keep you feeling full. Make sure that you fill yourself up with all this before having some dessert. Your meal should be rich in protein, dietary fats, and fiber.

What are the side effects of this diet?

There aren't any serious side effects of this diet that you should be worried about. You might feel light-headed and might experience mild headaches. However, this is a sign that your body is getting used to intermittent fasting and it isn't something that you should be worried about. Always make sure that your body is thoroughly hydrated. One more thing that you should keep in your mind is - always listen to your body. If you are feeling hungry before your fasting period ends, it is perfectly okay. Don't beat yourself up about it. Break your fast and eat something. Your body knows when it needs food, and it is good to listen to it. Don't think of this as a major setback. Instead, treat it as an isolated incident, and you can get back to your diet from the following day. Don't be too hard on yourself.

How long does it take to get used to fasting?

It will take your body a week or two to get used to intermittent fasting. Once your body gets used to this method of dieting, you can resume your exercising schedule. Make sure that your exercising schedule isn't too stressful during the first two weeks.

What are the benefits of this diet?

Fasting has many benefits to offer that go well beyond weight loss. Fasting can help in improving your overall health and improve the longevity of your life as well. In a recent study that was conducted to study the link between cell metabolism and fasting, it was found that fasting periodically can help in decreasing the risk of heart diseases, diabetes, aging, and so on. Fasting is effective because, during this period, a lot of cells that are present in the body die and the stem cells start working. This starts the regeneration process and produces new cells. Other studies also show that it helps in reducing the amount of bad cholesterol or LDL present in the blood.

How to keep hunger at bay while following this diet?

If you have just started your intermittent diet, you will probably have trouble trying to curb your thoughts about hunger. You may sit around and begin to wonder about how hungry you are and will probably crave for some form of food. So, let me give you a certain pattern that you could use during the first few days of your fast! Right before the first few hours of your fast, you should consume a huge meal! A huge meal, let us call it a monster meal. You will stop worrying about when you are going to eat next! You could try sleeping a decent amount of time since you cannot worry about hunger when you are dreaming! Try to keep yourself busy during the day to avoid worrying about your hunger. Last, but never the least, keep telling yourself that you do not need to think about hunger since you are a strong person!

Is it okay to consume certain beverages while fasting?

Yes, you can have certain beverages while fasting. However, make sure that there aren't any added calories in these drinks.

So, that means you will have to stay away from sodas and all sugary drinks. You can have calorie-free drinks like green tea, herbal teas, black coffee, or pretty much anything that doesn't have any calories in it. Make sure that you are drinking plenty of water and that your body is thoroughly hydrated. Watch out for the extra calories in milk and sugar. It might seem like a tough call to drink your morning coffee back, but you will get used to it, especially when you start to see the benefits of your intermittent fasting regime kicking in. Adding a bit of cream here, a spot of sugar there or even a bit of honey can have the effect of breaking the fast and sending your insulin levels back up. That means your body is not getting the full benefit of the fast. If you are doing a 24 hour fast, keep in mind that this is only for one or two days of the week so be strong about it and push on. If you are keen on losing weight, then you should stay away from alcohol. Alcohol is rich in calories, and it leads to unnecessary calorie consumption. If you feel like drinking, then stick to clear spirits or a glass of dry red or white wines. But that's about it. Don't overindulge in alcohol because this just prevents the process of weight loss.

Can intermittent fasting be combined with any other diet?

Intermittent fasting is one of the most versatile dieting protocols ever, and it can be easily clubbed with other diets like the ketogenic diet and the Paleo diet. A ketogenic diet is a low-carb and a high-fat diet in which the body produces ketones for providing energy and hence its name. The body produces ketones when there is a reduction in the consumption of carbs. When the carb consumption reduces, the body reaches into its reserves of fat for producing energy.

Intermittent fasting protocols can be easily combined with the ketogenic diet. You just need to make sure that during the eating window, the food that you are consuming has a high-fat content and low or no carbs in it. By combining intermittent fasting with any other dieting protocol, you can speed up the process of weight loss. Another diet that intermittent fasting can be effectively combined with is the Paleo diet. Paleo diet is a low-carb and a high-fat diet like the ketogenic diet. However, while following the Paleo diet, you will be allowed to eat only such foods that our Paleolithic ancestors could consume. This diet prohibits the consumption of all grains, processed foods, sugar, and anything that human beings produce by making use of machines. By being mindful of the food that you are consuming, you can make your weight-loss more effective.

Who shouldn't fast?

Certain people are expressly forbidden from following the intermittent fasting methods. Pregnant women and those who are breastfeeding should not follow these dieting protocols. If you suffer from bouts of weakness, are malnourished, anemic, frail, or exhausted, then in such a case, you shouldn't fast.

Consult a doctor before fasting if you happen to have any medical condition. If you are dependent on any medication, have a weak immune system, high blood pressure, or a weak circulation then consult your doctor. If you have any eating disorders like anorexia or bulimia, you shouldn't fast. Fasting will just worsen these conditions. If you have undergone any major surgery recently, or are recovering from any major illness, then in such a case you definitely shouldn't fast. Fasting before a major surgery is forbidden too.

Conclusion

By now you would have understood what intermittent fasting is all about. Fasting for prolonged periods of time can help you to achieve your weight loss goals while improving your overall health. Intermittent fasting is a flexible diet, and you can customize it according to your convenience and needs. There are plenty of benefits this diet offers, and you can reap all these benefits by adjusting your pattern of eating. Two of the most popular variations of this diet are the 16/8 method and the 24-hour fasting protocol. Select a method according to your daily schedule. By incorporating some form of exercising into your daily schedule, you can build lean muscle while following this diet.

Thank you for purchasing this book, I hope you enjoyed it.

Finally, if you enjoyed this book then I'd like to ask you for a favor. Will you be kind enough to leave a review for this book on Amazon? It would be greatly appreciated!

Don't forget to follow us on Twitter, Facebook & Instagram to get empowered, educated and inspired to become the best version of yourself in life! You deserve it.

Thank you and good luck!